The Definitive Mediterranean Diet Cookbook

A Comprehensive Set of Life changing Mediterranean Diet Recipes for Rapid Weight Loss

Georgette Poe

Table of Contents

INTRODUCTION

I've put together a long weekly sample schedule below to help you work through some balanced Mediterranean diet recipes and look forward to a healthy week of meal planning at the beginning of the week. While this meal is not a typical Greek dish, it is a delicious Mediterranean dish. Orthodox Mediterranean Diet Plans outline all of the things that people in the Mediterranean consume in their everyday lives. A chicken dish that only needs a few ingredients and is perfect for the Mediterranean diet.

You can make them with almost any meal from a typical Mediterranean diet if you pay attention to the ingredients. However, I recommend that you look at the Greek dietary recommendations, which basically reflect the Mediterranean diet's variety of portions.

If you follow a Mediterranean diet, you'll be able to eat a variety of filling meals like greens, soups, burgers, and salads. Eat a variety of vegetables, including those that resemble white beans, as well as fruits and vegetables.

Here you'll find everything from fish salads to cereals and everything in between if you're searching for any Mediterranean lunch recipes to get you through the week. These filling and tasty lunches will help you stick to a Mediterranean diet for the rest of the day.

Check out this collection of recipes that combine the best of the Mediterranean diet's ingredients, including fresh fruits, herbs, cereals, almonds, legumes, spices, and more.

Mediterranean dishes are a perfect addition to every menu because of their vivid flavors and vibrant items. Plant foods such as nuts, potatoes, legumes, fruits, onions, nuts, and more are included in this balanced Mediterranean recipe. These Mediterranean diet recipes are only a small sample of the countless typical Mediterranean recipes available. Every week is a winner with our beginner's cookbook to Mediterranean cuisine, which includes basic tips and recipes that are weekday-friendly, child-friendly, and perfect for your family.

We consider having seafood about twice a week in our Mediterranean diet, which focuses on a balanced and healthy solution. Since our recipes are all vegetable-based, it's important to include seafood, as well as other Mediterranean foods like grains, beans, legumes, fruits, tomatoes, nuts, and more, in your seafood diet. With our cookbook to the best ideas for a balanced, healthy lifestyle, we help you learn the Mediterranean diet.

The following recipes are ideal for enjoying right now because they are full of nutritious, healthy, and tasty Mediterranean food ideas for the Mediterranean diet. This grilled chicken is sure to become one of your favorite Mediterranean recipes. The Food and Drug Administration (FDA) and the European Food Safety Authority (EFSA) have also approved a pan of salmon (EFSA).

The Mediterranean diet doesn't allow for much mayonnaise, but this salad makes up for it because it's the rich, creamy carrot salad you're after. Instead of the usual pasta salad, any who want to save time should go for a cereal salad. Since the Mediterranean diet consists solely of carbs and allows for the consumption of pasta, this salad is ideal for those occasions when you need a break.

The Mediterranean diet aims to provide you with nutritious, tasty meals that encourage you to spend less time at the kitchen table and more time with your family. If you're interested in testing out this nutritious and common lifestyle, here are some tips to get you started, as well as some of the long-term benefits you might reap if you stick to it. The standard Mediterranean diet, which includes the same menu as mine, is described below. I've included some of my favorite Mediterranean dish ideas from the last few years below.

I will certainly re-edit some of the special Mediterranean recipes that I have never used before. I've made a recipe card for each recipe, which you can find below, as well as a list of some of my favorite recipes from the past few years.

Before we get through the rundown of Mediterranean diet recipes, let me cover a few basics if you're new to Mediterranean cuisine. In this post, I define the "Mediterranean Diet" and provide a seven-day diet plan for people. Here are a few short directions for you if you either don't know where to begin or are simply overwhelmed by all

the choices. I struggled to choose only a few ingredients for
the Mediterranean diet, but there's so much more to enjoy.

BREAKFAST RECIPES

1. Leeks and Eggs Muffins

Preparation time: 10 minutes

Cooking time: 20 minutes

Servings: 2

Ingredients:

- 3 eggs, whisked
- ¼ cup baby spinach
- 2 tablespoons leeks, chopped
- 4 tablespoons parmesan, grated
- 2 tablespoons almond milk
- Cooking spray
- 1 small red bell pepper, chopped
- Salt and black pepper to the taste
- 1 tomato, cubed
- 2 tablespoons cheddar cheese, grated

Directions:

1. In a bowl, combine the eggs with the milk, salt, pepper and the rest of the ingredients except the cooking spray and whisk well.
2. Grease a muffin tin with the cooking spray and divide the eggs mixture in each muffin mould.

3. Bake at 380 degrees F for 20 minutes and serve them for breakfast.

Nutrition: calories 308, fat 19.4, fiber 1.7, carbs 8.7, protein 24.4

2. Artichokes and Cheese Omelet

Preparation time: 10 minutes

Cooking time: 8 minutes

Servings: 1

Ingredients:

- 1 teaspoon avocado oil
- 1 tablespoon almond milk
- 2 eggs, whisked
- A pinch of salt and black pepper
- 2 tablespoons tomato, cubed
- 2 tablespoons kalamata olives, pitted and sliced
- 1 artichoke heart, chopped
- 1 tablespoon tomato sauce
- 1 tablespoon feta cheese, crumbled

Directions:

1. In a bowl, combine the eggs with the milk, salt, pepper and the rest of the ingredients except the avocado oil and whisk well.

2. Heat up a pan with the avocado oil over medium-high heat, add the omelet mix, spread into the pan, cook for 4 minutes, flip, cook for 4 minutes more, transfer to a plate and serve.

Nutrition: calories 303, fat 17.7, fiber 9.9, carbs 21.9, protein 18.2

3. Quinoa and Eggs Salad

Preparation time: 5 minutes

Cooking time: 0 minutes

Servings: 4

Ingredients:

- 4 eggs, soft boiled, peeled and cut into wedges
- 2 cups baby arugula
- 2 cups cherry tomatoes, halved
- 1 cucumber, sliced
- 1 cup quinoa, cooked
- 1 cup almonds, chopped
- 1 avocado, peeled, pitted and sliced
- 1 tablespoon olive oil
- ½ cup mixed dill and mint, chopped
- A pinch of salt and black pepper
- Juice of 1 lemon

Directions:

1. In a large salad bowl, combine the eggs with the arugula and the rest of the ingredients, toss, divide between plates and serve for breakfast.

Nutrition: calories 519, fat 32.4, fiber 11, carbs 43.3, protein 19.1

4. Corn and Shrimp Salad

Preparation time: 10 minutes

Cooking time: 10 minutes

Servings: 4

Ingredients:

- 4 ears of sweet corn, husked
- 1 avocado, peeled, pitted and chopped
- ½ cup basil, chopped
- A pinch of salt and black pepper
- 1-pound shrimp, peeled and deveined
- 1 and ½ cups cherry tomatoes, halved
- ¼ cup olive oil

Directions:

1. Put the corn in a pot, add water to cover, bring to a boil over medium heat, cook for 6 minutes, drain, cool down, cut corn from the cob and put it in a bowl.
2. Thread the shrimp onto skewers and brush with some of the oil.

3. Place the skewers on the preheated grill, cook over medium heat for 2 minutes on each side, remove from skewers and add over the corn.

4. Add the rest of the ingredients to the bowl, toss, divide between plates and serve for breakfast.

Nutrition: calories 371, fat 22, fiber 5, carbs 25, protein 23

5. Tomato and Lentils Salad

Preparation time: 10 minutes

Cooking time: 35 minutes

Servings: 4

Ingredients:

- 2 yellow onions, chopped
- 4 garlic cloves, minced
- 2 cups brown lentils
- 1 tablespoon olive oil
- A pinch of salt and black pepper
- ½ teaspoon sweet paprika
- ½ teaspoon ginger, grated
- 3 cups water
- ¼ cup lemon juice
- ¾ cup Greek yogurt
- 3 tablespoons tomato paste

Directions:

1. Heat up a pot with the oil over medium-high heat, add the onions and sauté for 2 minutes.
2. Add the garlic and the lentils, stir and cook for 1 minute more.
3. Add the water, bring to a simmer and cook covered for 30 minutes.

4. Add the lemon juice and the remaining ingredients except the yogurt. toss, divide the mix into bowls, top with the yogurt and serve.

Nutrition: calories 294, fat 3, fiber 8, carbs 49, protein 21

6. Couscous and Chickpeas Bowls

Preparation time: 10 minutes

Cooking time: 6 minutes

Servings: 4

Ingredients:

- ¾ cup whole wheat couscous
- 1 yellow onion, chopped
- 1 tablespoon olive oil
- 1 cup water
- 2 garlic cloves, minced
- 15 ounces canned chickpeas, drained and rinsed
- A pinch of salt and black pepper
- 15 ounces canned tomatoes, chopped
- 14 ounces canned artichokes, drained and chopped
- ½ cup Greek olives, pitted and chopped
- ½ teaspoon oregano, dried
- 1 tablespoon lemon juice

Directions:

1. Put the water in a pot, bring to a boil over medium heat, add the couscous, stir, take off the heat, cover the pan, leave aside for 10 minutes and fluff with a fork.
2. Heat up a pan with the oil over medium-high heat, add the onion and sauté for 2 minutes.
3. Add the rest of the ingredients, toss and cook for 4 minutes more.

4. Add the couscous, toss, divide into bowls and serve for breakfast.

Nutrition: calories 340, fat 10, fiber 9, carbs 51, protein 11

7. Zucchini and Quinoa Pan

Preparation time: 10 minutes

Cooking time: 20 minutes

Servings: 4

Ingredients:

- 1 tablespoon olive oil
- 2 garlic cloves, minced
- 1 cup quinoa
- 1 zucchini, roughly cubed
- 2 tablespoons basil, chopped
- ¼ cup green olives, pitted and chopped
- 1 tomato, cubed
- ½ cup feta cheese, crumbled
- 2 cups water
- 1 cup canned garbanzo beans, drained and rinsed
- A pinch of salt and black pepper

Directions:

1. Heat up a pan with the oil over medium-high heat, add the garlic and quinoa and brown for 3 minutes.
2. Add the water, zucchinis, salt and pepper, toss, bring to a simmer and cook for 15 minutes.
3. Add the rest of the ingredients, toss, divide everything between plates and serve for breakfast.

Nutrition: calories 310, fat 11, fiber 6, carbs 42, protein 11

LUNCH RECIPES

8. Pumpkin Soup with Rice and Spinach

Preparation Time: 15 minutes

Cooking Time: 15 minutes

Servings: 2

Ingredients:

- 3 small pumpkins, concerning one pound
- 2 tablespoons extra virgin olive oil
- medium onion, chopped
- leek, white half only
- medium potatoes, bare-assed and diced
- cups vegetable stock or water
- cups milk
- 1 bay leaf
- A sprig of thyme
- A grating of nutmeg
- Salt
- Freshly ground black pepper
- cup Arborio rice
- 2-pound spinach
- tablespoons butter
- Freshly grated Parmesan cheese

Directions

1. Slice the pumpkin. stop the skin and take away the seeds and pith.
2. Dice the flesh into little items. Heat the vegetable oil in an exceedingly massive cooking pan and cook the onion and leek over a moderate heat till they're softened.
3. Add the pumpkin, potatoes, stock or water, milk, and herbs and produce to a boil. cowl and simmer for 30 minutes or till the vegetables are tender. Season with nutmeg, salt, and black pepper.
4. Remove the herb and thyme. You should force it via a sieve or puree in an exceedingly liquidizer.
5. Return to the pot, adding a touch a lot of water if the soup is simply too thick. Rouse a boil.
6. Add the rice and cook for twenty a lot of minutes or till the rice is tender but still firm.
7. Meanwhile, wash the spinach carefully and cook in an exceedingly lined pan over a moderate heat for five minutes or till it is simply tender. Drain well and chop coarsely.
8. Melt 1/2 the butter in an exceedingly cooking pan and cook the spinach over a delicate heat for three or four minutes.
9. Augment the soup. Stir within the remaining butter and serve hot with cheese on the facet.

Nutrition: Calories: 123, Fats: 3g, Dietary Fiber: 5g, Carbohydrates: 19g, Protein: 5g

9. Nettle Soup

Preparation Time: 15 minutes

Cooking Time: 15 minutes

Servings: 2

Ingredients:

- 6 ounces nettles
- 3 tablespoons further virgin olive oil
- 2 medium onions, sliced
- pound potatoes, bare-assed and diced
- 5 cups water
- cup crème fraiche
- Salt
- Freshly ground black pepper

Directions

1. Wash the nettles fastidiously and put aside.
2. Heat the olive oil in an exceedingly massive cooking pan and cook the onions over a moderate heat for five minutes.
3. Add the nettles, potatoes, and water, and produce to a boil.
4. Cover and simmer for half-hour. Force through a sieve or puree in an exceedingly liquidizer.
5. Return to the cooking pan and warmth totally.
6. Stir within the crème fraiche and after that you should Season it with salt & black pepper.

Nutrition: 195 Calories 9.6g Fat 7.6g Protein

10. Wild Mushroom Soup

Preparation Time: 15 minutes

Cooking Time: 15 minutes

Servings: 2

Ingredients:

- pound mixed wild mushrooms
- 4 tablespoons further virgin olive oil
- Spanish onion, chopped
- ripe plum tomatoes, peeled, seeded, and chopped
- 5 cups vegetable broth or water
- Salt
- Freshly ground black pepper
- FOR THE PICADA:
- 15 blanched almonds
- slice white bread concerning one in. thick (crust removed)
- 1-2 tablespoons further virgin olive oil
- garlic cloves, crushed
- Pinch of saffron powder

Directions

1. To build the soup, wash the mushrooms fastidiously and wipe dry.
2. Cut them into three or four items consistent with their size and heat the vegetable oil

3. In an exceedingly massive pan and cook the onion over a delicate heat for concerning ten minutes or till it starts to show golden.
4. Add the tomatoes and still cook till any liquid is gaseous and also the tomatoes are reduced to a pulp.
5. Stir within the mushrooms.
6. Cowl and simmer for quarter-hour, stirring from time to time therefore the mushrooms cook equally.
7. You should add the broth & convey to a boil. Simmer, uncovered, for twenty minutes. After that you should Season it with salt & black pepper.
8. To build the picada, toast the almonds in an exceedingly 350°F kitchen appliance until they're golden chop coarsely.
9. Heat one or a pair of tablespoons vegetable oil in an exceedingly small cooking pan.
10. And fry the bread till it's golden on each side drain on a paper towel and withdraw little items or Crush or grind the almonds, deep-fried bread, garlic, and saffron with a mortar and pestle
11. In an exceedingly kitchen appliance, till all the ingredients type a sleek, thick paste.
12. Mix with a tablespoon or 2 of the soup into the picada, then stir the mixture into the soup.
13. Place a slice of bread on the lowest of 4 man or woman soup bowls. Pour the new soup over the bread and serve.

Nutrition: 195 Calories 9.6g Fat 7.6g Protein

11. Tomato and Alimentary Paste Soup

Preparation Time: 15 minutes

Cooking Time: 15 minutes

Servings: 2

Ingredients:

- 3 tablespoons further virgin olive oil
- massive onion, chopped
- garlic cloves, finely chopped
- 1-2 red chili peppers, cored, seeded, and finely chopped
- cup canned plum tomatoes, forced through a sieve or pureed in a food processor
- bunch Petroselinum crispum, finely chopped
- 6 cups water
- ounces fine alimentary paste or (angel hair)
- Salt

Directions

1. Heat the vegetable oil in an exceedingly massive pot and cook the onion over moderate heat till it's softened.
2. Add the garlic and chili peppers and cook for two a lot of minutes.
3. Add the tomato puree and parsley and cook for a further five minutes.
4. Pour within the water and produce to a boil. Simmer for ten minutes.

5. Increase the warmth. Once the soup is boiling, come by the alimentary paste and cook till it's tender however still firm.

6. Finally, you need to Season it with salt and serve hot.

Nutrition: Calories: 123, Fats: 3g, Dietary Fiber: 5g, Carbohydrates: 19g, Protein: 5g

12. Sorrel Soup

Preparation Time: 15 minutes

Cooking Time: 15 minutes

Servings: 2

Ingredients:

- 1-pound sorrel
- 3 tablespoons butter
- 3 tablespoons flour
- 5 cups quandary (or .05 water and half milk)
- A grating of nutmeg
- Salt
- Freshly ground black pepper

Directions

1. Wash the sorrel fastidiously and take away the stalks and larger ribs.
2. Heat the butter in an exceedingly massive cooking pan and add the sorrel.
3. Cover and cook over a delicate heat till the sorrel has softened into a puree.
4. Stir within the flour and cook for two minutes.
5. Gradually add the new water, stirring perpetually, till the soup is slightly thickened.
6. Simmer for twenty minutes. Finally, you must season it with nutmeg, salt, and black pepper.

Nutrition: Calories: 123, Fats: 3g, Dietary Fiber: 5g, Carbohydrates: 19g, Protein: 5g

13. Summer Vegetable Soup

Preparation Time: 15 minutes

Cooking Time: 15 minutes

Servings: 2

Ingredients:

- medium eggplant (about ~ pound)
- pound zucchini
- red, green, or yellow bell peppers
- cup further virgin olive oil
- massive onion, thinly sliced
- celery stalks, diced
- pound waxy potatoes, peeled and diced
- 2-pound ripe plum tomatoes, peeled, seeded, and chopped
- cups water
- 2 tablespoons torn basil leaves
- Salt
- Freshly ground black pepper
- Freshly grated pecorino or Parmesan cheese

Directions

1. Peel and dice the eggplant. Trim the ends of the zucchini and withdraw rounds.
2. Cut the peppers into quarters and take away the cores and seeds. withdraw skinny strips and heat the vegetable oil

3. In an exceedingly massive pot and cook the onion, celery, and potatoes over a coffee heat for ten minutes

4. Stirring from time to time therefore the vegetables cook equally.

5. Add the eggplant, zucchini, and peppers, cover, and cook for an additional ten minutes.

6. Add the tomatoes and cook, uncovered, for 10 more minutes.

7. Pour within the water and produce to a boil.

8. Cowl and simmer for fifteen to 20 minutes or till the vegetables are tender.

9. The soup ought to be terribly thick, almost a stew.

10. Add the basil and simmer for two or three minutes.

11. After that you should Season it with salt & black pepper. Serve hot with cheese on the facet.

Nutrition: Calories: 123, Fats: 3g, Dietary Fiber: 5g, Carbohydrates: 19g, Protein: 5g

14. Tuscan Black Cabbage Soup

Preparation Time: 15 minutes

Cooking Time: 15 minutes

Servings: 2

Ingredients:

- pound Tuscan black cabbage
- tablespoons further virgin olive oil
- large onion, thinly sliced
- celery stalk, thinly sliced
- carrot, diced
- medium potato, bare-assed and diced
- 5 cups vegetable broth or water
- Salt
- Freshly ground black pepper
- slices wheaten bread
- garlic cloves, peeled, and cut in half
- Freshly grated Parmesan cheese

Directions

1. Wash the cabbage and take away the stalks. Withdraw skinny strips and heat the vegetable oil
2. in an exceedingly massive pot and cook the onion, celery, carrot, and potato for three minutes.
3. Add the cabbage and broth and bring to a boil cowl and simmer for one hour and you should After that you should Season it with salt & black pepper.

4. Meanwhile place the slices of bread on a baking receptacle and toast

5. In an exceedingly preheated 375 ·p kitchen appliance till they're golden.

6. Take away from the kitchen appliance and rub every slice with garlic.

7. Place the slices of bread into individual soup bowls and pour the new soup over them.

8. Serve at once with cheese on the facet.

DINNER RECIPES

15. Medi Sausage with Rice

Preparation Time: 15 minutes

Cooking Time 8 hours

Servings: 6

Ingredients

- 1½ pounds Italian sausage, crumbled
- 1 medium onion, chopped
- 2 tablespoons steak sauce
- 2 cups long grain rice, uncooked
- 1 (14-ounce) can diced tomatoes with juice
- ½ cup water
- 1 medium green pepper, diced

Directions

1. Spray your slow cooker with olive oil or nonstick cooking spray. Add the sausage, onion, and steak sauce to the slow cooker. Put on low for 9 hours.
2. After 8 hours, add the rice, tomatoes, water and green pepper. Stir to combine thoroughly. Cook an additional 20 to 25 minutes.

Nutrition: 650 Calories 36g Fat 11g Carbohydrates 22g Protein

16. Albondigas

Preparation Time: 20 minutes

Cooking Time 5 hours

Servings: 6

Ingredients

- 1-pound ground turkey
- 1-pound ground pork
- 2 eggs
- 1 (20-ounce) can diced tomatoes
- ¾ cup sweet onion, minced, divided
- ¼ cup plus 1 tablespoon breadcrumbs
- 3 tablespoons fresh parsley, chopped
- 1½ teaspoons cumin
- 1½ teaspoons paprika (sweet or hot)

Directions

1. Spray the slow cooker with olive oil.
2. In a mixing bowl, incorporate the ground meat, eggs, about half of the onions, the breadcrumbs, and the spices.
3. Wash your hands and mix together until everything is well combined. Do not over-mix, though, as this makes for tough meatballs. Shape into meatballs. How big you make them will obviously determine how many total meatballs you get.

4. In a skillet, cook 2 tablespoons of olive oil over medium heat. Once hot, mix in the meatballs and brown on all sides. Make sure the balls aren't touching each other so they brown evenly. Once done, transfer them to the slow cooker.

5. Add the rest of the onions and the tomatoes to the skillet and allow them to cook for a few minutes, scraping the brown bits from the meatballs up to add flavor. Transfer the tomatoes over the meatballs in the slow cooker and cook on low for 5 hours.

Nutrition: 372 Calories 21.7g Fat 15g Carbohydrates 28.6 Protein

17. Baked Bean Fish Meal

Preparation Time: 10 minutes

Cooking Time: 10 minutes

Servings: 4

Ingredients:

- 1 tablespoon balsamic vinegar
- 2 ½ cups green beans
- 1-pint cherry or grape tomatoes
- 4 (4-ounce each) fish fillets, such as cod or tilapia
- 2 tablespoons olive oil

Directions:

1. Preheat an oven to 400 degrees. Grease two baking sheets with some olive oil or olive oil spray. Arrange 2 fish fillets on each sheet. In a mixing bowl, pour olive oil and vinegar. Combine to mix well with each other.
2. Mix green beans and tomatoes. Combine to mix well with each other. Combine both mixtures well with each other. Add mixture equally over fish fillets. Bake for 6-8 minutes, until fish opaque and easy to flake. Serve warm.

Nutrition: 229 Calories 13g Fat 2.5g Protein

18. Mushroom Cod Stew

Preparation Time: 10 minutes

Cooking Time: 20 minutes

Servings: 6

Ingredients:

- 2 tablespoons extra-virgin olive oil
- 2 garlic cloves, minced
- 1 can tomato
- 2 cups chopped onion
- ¾ teaspoon smoked paprika
- a (12-ounce) jar roasted red peppers
- 1/3 cup dry red wine
- ¼ teaspoon kosher or sea salt
- ¼ teaspoon black pepper
- 1 cup black olives
- 1 ½ pounds cod fillets, cut into 1-inch pieces
- 3 cups sliced mushrooms

Directions:

1. Get medium-large cooking pot, warm up oil over medium heat. Add onions and stir-cook for 4 minutes.
2. Add garlic and smoked paprika; cook for 1 minute, stirring often. Add tomatoes with juice, roasted peppers, olives, wine, pepper, and salt; stir gently.

3. Boil mixture. Add the cod and mushrooms; turn down heat to medium. Close and cook until the cod is easy to flake, stir in between. Serve warm.

Nutrition: 238 Calories 7g Fat 3.5g Protein

19. Spiced Swordfish

Preparation Time: 10 minutes

Cooking Time: 15 minutes

Servings: 4

Ingredients:

- 4 (7 ounces each) swordfish steaks
- 1/2 teaspoon ground black pepper
- 12 cloves of garlic, peeled
- 3/4 teaspoon salt
- 1 1/2 teaspoon ground cumin
- 1 teaspoon paprika
- 1 teaspoon coriander
- 3 tablespoons lemon juice
- 1/3 cup olive oil

Directions:

1. Using food processor, incorporate all the ingredients excluding for swordfish. Secure the lid and blend until smooth mixture. Pat dry fish steaks; coat equally with the prepared spice mixture.
2. Situate them over an aluminum foil, cover and refrigerator for 1 hour. Prep a griddle pan over high heat, pour oil and heat it. Stir in fish steaks; stir-cook for 5-6 minutes per side. Serve warm.

Nutrition: 255 Calories 12g Fat 0.5g Protein

20. Anchovy Pasta Mania

Preparation Time: 10 minutes

Cooking Time: 20 minutes

Servings: 4

Ingredients:

- 4 anchovy fillets, packed in olive oil
- ½ pound broccoli, cut into 1-inch florets
- 2 cloves garlic, sliced
- 1-pound whole-wheat penne
- 2 tablespoons olive oil
- ¼ cup Parmesan cheese, grated
- Salt and black pepper, to taste
- Red pepper flakes, to taste

Directions:

1. Cook pasta as directed over pack; drain and set aside. Take a medium saucepan or skillet, add oil. Heat over medium heat.
2. Add anchovies, broccoli, and garlic, and stir-cook until veggies turn tender for 4-5 minutes. Take off heat; mix in the pasta. Serve warm with Parmesan cheese, red pepper flakes, salt, and black pepper sprinkled on top.

Nutrition: 328 Calories 8g Fat 7g Protein

21. Shrimp Garlic Pasta

Preparation Time: 10 minutes

Cooking Time: 15 minutes

Servings: 4

Ingredients:

- 1-pound shrimp
- 3 garlic cloves, minced
- 1 onion, finely chopped
- 1 package whole wheat or bean pasta
- 4 tablespoons olive oil
- Salt and black pepper, to taste
- ¼ cup basil, cut into strips
- ¾ cup chicken broth, low-sodium

Directions:

1. Cook pasta as directed over pack; rinse and set aside. Get medium saucepan, add oil then warm up over medium heat. Add onion, garlic and stir-cook until become translucent and fragrant for 3 minutes.
2. Add shrimp, black pepper (ground) and salt; stir-cook for 3 minutes until shrimps are opaque. Add broth and simmer for 2-3 more minutes. Add pasta in serving plates; add shrimp mixture over; serve warm with basil on top.

Nutrition: 605 Calories 17g Fat 19g Protein

MEAT RECIPES

22. Chives Chicken and Radishes

Preparation time: 10 minutes

Cooking time: 30 minutes

Servings: 4

Ingredients:

- 2 chicken breasts, skinless, boneless and cubed
- Salt and black pepper to the taste
- 1 tablespoon olive oil
- 1 cup chicken stock
- ½ cup tomato sauce
- ½ pound red radishes, cubed
- 2 tablespoon chives, chopped

Directions:

1. Heat up a Dutch oven with the oil over medium-high heat, add the chicken and brown for 4 minutes on each side.
2. Add the rest of the ingredients except the chives, bring to a simmer and cook over medium heat for 20 minutes.
3. Divide the mix between plates, sprinkle the chives on top and serve.

Nutrition: calories 277, fat 15, fiber 9.3, carbs 20.9, protein 33.2

23. Feta Chicken and Cabbage

Preparation time: 10 minutes

Cooking time: 25 minutes

Servings: 4

Ingredients:

- 2 chicken breasts, skinless, boneless and cut into strips
- 1 red cabbage, shredded
- 2 tablespoons olive oil
- Salt and black pepper to the taste
- 2 tablespoons balsamic vinegar
- 1 and ½ cups tomatoes, cubed
- 1 tablespoon chives, chopped
- ¼ cup feta cheese, crumbled

Directions:

1. Heat up a pan with the oil over medium-high heat, add the chicken and brown for 5 minutes.
2. Add the rest of the ingredients except the cheese, and cook over medium heat for 20 minutes stirring often.
3. Add the cheese, toss, divide everything between plates and serve.

Nutrition: calories 277, fat 15, fiber 8.6, carbs 14.9, protein 14.2

24. Garlic Chicken and Endives

Preparation time: 10 minutes

Cooking time: 15 minutes

Servings: 4

Ingredients:

- 1-pound chicken breasts, skinless, boneless and cubed
- 2 endives, sliced
- 2 tablespoons olive oil
- 4 garlic cloves, minced
- ½ cup chicken stock
- 2 tablespoons parmesan, grated
- 1 tablespoon parsley, chopped
- Salt and black pepper to the taste

Directions:

1. Heat up a pan with the oil over medium-high heat, add the chicken and cook for 5 minutes.
2. Add the endives, garlic, the stock, salt and pepper, stir, bring to a simmer and cook over medium-high heat for 10 minutes.
3. Add the parmesan and the parsley, toss gently, divide everything between plates and serve.

Nutrition: calories 280, fat 9.2, fiber 10.8, carbs 21.6, protein 33.8

25. Brown Rice, Chicken and Scallions

Preparation time: 10 minutes

Cooking time: 30 minutes

Servings: 4

Ingredients:

- 1 and ½ cups brown rice
- 3 cups chicken stock
- 2 tablespoon balsamic vinegar
- 1-pound chicken breast, boneless, skinless and cubed
- 6 scallions, chopped
- Salt and black pepper to the taste
- 1 tablespoon sweet paprika
- 2 tablespoons avocado oil

Directions:

1. Heat up a pan with the oil over medium-high heat, add the chicken and brown for 5 minutes.
2. Add the scallions and sauté for 5 minutes more.
3. Add the rice and the rest of the ingredients, bring to a simmer and cook over medium heat for 20 minutes.
4. Stir the mix, divide everything between plates and serve.

Nutrition: calories 300, fat 9.2, fiber 11.8, carbs 18.6, protein 23.8

26. Creamy Chicken and Mushrooms

Preparation time: 10 minutes

Cooking time: 30 minutes

Servings: 4

Ingredients:

- 1 red onion, chopped
- 1 tablespoon olive oil
- 2 garlic cloves, minced
- 2 carrots chopped
- Salt and black pepper to the taste
- 1 tablespoon thyme, chopped
- 1 and ½ cups chicken stock
- ½ pound Bella mushrooms, sliced
- 1 cup heavy cream
- 2 chicken breasts, skinless, boneless and cubed
- 2 tablespoons chives, chopped
- 1 tablespoon parsley, chopped

Directions:

1. Heat up a Dutch oven with the oil over medium-high heat, add the onion and the garlic and sauté for 5 minutes.
2. Add the chicken and the mushrooms, and sauté for 10 minutes more.

3. Add the rest of the ingredients except the chives and the parsley, bring to a simmer and cook over medium heat for 15 minutes.
4. Add the chives and parsley, divide the mix between plates and serve.

Nutrition: calories 275, fat 11.9, fiber 10.6, carbs 26.7, protein 23.7

27. Curry Chicken, Artichokes and Olives

Preparation time: 5 minutes

Cooking time: 7 hours

Servings: 6

Ingredients:

- 2 pounds chicken breasts, boneless, skinless and cubed
- 12 ounces canned artichoke hearts, drained
- 1 cup chicken stock
- 1 red onion, chopped
- 1 tablespoon white wine vinegar
- 1 cup kalamata olives, pitted and chopped
- 1 tablespoon curry powder
- 2 teaspoons basil, dried
- Salt and black pepper to the taste
- ¼ cup rosemary, chopped

Directions:

1. In your slow cooker, combine the chicken with the artichokes, olives and the rest of the ingredients, put the lid on and cook on Low for 7 hours.
2. Divide the mix between plates and serve hot.

Nutrition: calories 275, fat 11.9, fiber 7.6, carbs 19.7, protein 18.7

28. Slow Cooked Chicken and Capers Mix

Preparation time: 5 minutes

Cooking time: 7 hours

Servings: 4

Ingredients:

- 2 chicken breasts, skinless, boneless and halved
- 2 cups canned tomatoes, crushed
- 2 garlic cloves, minced
- 1 yellow onion, chopped
- 2 cups chicken stock
- 2 tablespoons capers, drained
- ¼ cup rosemary, chopped
- Salt and black pepper to the taste

Directions:

1. In your slow cooker, combine the chicken with the tomatoes, capers and the rest of the ingredients, put the lid on and cook on Low for 7 hours.
2. Divide the mix between plates and serve.

Nutrition: calories 292, fat 9.4, fiber 11.8, carbs 25.1, protein 36.4

SIDE DISH AND PIZZA RECIPES

29. Ideal Pizza Dough (On A Large Baking Sheet)

Preparation Time: 10 minutes

Cooking Time: 1 hour

Servings: 5

Ingredients:

- Wheat flour 13 oz.
- Salt 1.5 tsp.
- Dry yeast 1,799 tsp.
- Sugar 1 tsp.
- Water 200 ml
- 1 tbsp. olive oil
- Dried Basil 1.5 tsp.

Directions:

1. We cultivate yeast in warm water. There you can add a spoonful of sugar, so the yeast will begin to work faster. Leave them for 10 minutes.
2. Sift the flour through a sieve (leave 2 oz. for the future) in a deep bowl. Add salt, basil, mix. Pour water with yeast into the cavity in the flour and mix thoroughly with a fork.

3. Somewhere in the middle of the process, when the dough becomes less than one whole, add olive oil. When the dough is ready, cover with a damp towel and put in heat for 30 minutes.
4. Now just lay it on a flour dusted surface and roll out the future pizza to a thickness of 2-3 mm.
5. The main rule of pizza is the maximum possible temperature, minimum time. Therefore, feel free to set the highest temperature that is available in your oven.

Nutrition: Calories: 193 Protein: 10.3g Carbs: 34g Fat: 9.3g

30. Vegetable Oil Pizza Dough

Preparation Time: 10 minutes

Cooking Time: 1 hour

Servings: 3

Ingredients:

- Wheat flour 1 cup
- Water 1 cup
- Salt to taste
- Vegetable oil 1 tbsp.
- Dry yeast 10 g

Directions:

1. We mix water and yeast, leave for 40 minutes so that they disperse. You can add a tablespoon of sugar.
2. Then pour in the oil, add the flour; knead well and put in a warm place to increase the volume by 2 times.

Nutrition: Calories: 223 Protein: 10.3g Carbs: 9.4g Fat: 5.3g

31. Pizza Dough on Yogurt

Preparation Time: 10 minutes

Cooking Time: 30 minutes

Servings: 5

Ingredients:

- Natural yogurt 9 oz.
- Vegetable oil 5 tbsp.
- ½ tsp. salt
- Wheat flour 2.5 cups
- Baking powder 1 tsp.

Directions:

1. Mix flour, baking powder and salt. Add yogurt and butter, mix everything thoroughly. Preheat the oven to 190 ° C.
2. Lubricate the pan with oil. Roll the dough very thinly and transfer to a baking sheet. Put the filling to taste. Bake for 10-15 minutes.

Nutrition: Calories: 336 Protein: 10.3g Carbs: 24g Fat: 13.3g

32. Eggplant Pizza

Preparation Time: 10 minutes

Cooking Time: 30 minutes

Servings: 6

Ingredients:

- Eggplants (1 large or 2 medium)
- Olive oil (.33 cup)
- Black pepper & salt (as desired)
- Marinara sauce - store-bought/homemade (1.25 cups)
- Shredded mozzarella cheese (1.5 cups)
- Cherry tomatoes (2 cups - halved)
- Torn basil leaves (.5 cup)

Directions:

1. Heat the oven to reach 400°F. Prepare a baking sheet with a layer of parchment baking paper.
2. Slice the end/ends off of the eggplant and them it into ¾-inch slices. Arrange the slices on the prepared sheet and brush both sides with olive oil. Dust with pepper and salt to your liking.
3. Roast the eggplant until tender (10 to 12 min.).
4. Transfer the tray from the oven and add two tbsp. of sauce on top of each section. Top it off with the mozzarella and three to five tomato pieces on top.
5. Bake it until the cheese is melted. The tomatoes should begin to blister in about five to seven more

minutes. Take the tray from the oven. Serve hot and garnish with a dusting of basil.

Nutrition: Protein: 8 g Fat: 20 g Carbs: 25 g Calories: 257

33. Mediterranean Whole Wheat Pizza

Preparation Time: 5 minutes

Cooking Time: 25 minutes

Servings: 4

Ingredients:

- Whole-wheat pizza crust (1)
- Basil pesto (4 oz. jar)
- Artichoke hearts (.5 cup)
- Kalamata olives (2 tbsp.)
- Pepperoncini (2 tbsp. drained)
- Feta cheese (.25 cup)

Directions:

1. Program the oven to 450°F. Drain and pull the artichokes to pieces. Slice/chop the pepperoncini and olives.
2. Arrange the pizza crust onto a floured work surface and cover it using pesto. Arrange the artichoke, pepperoncini slices, and olives over the pizza. Lastly, crumble and add the feta.
3. Bake in the hot oven until the cheese has melted, and it has a crispy crust or 10-12 minutes.

Nutrition: Calories: 277 Protein: 9.7 g Carbs: 24 g Fat: 18.6 g

34. Fruit Pizza

Preparation time: 15 minutes

Cooking time: 0 minutes

Servings: 4

Ingredients:

- 4 watermelon slices
- 1 oz blueberries
- 2 oz goat cheese, crumbled
- 1 teaspoon fresh parsley, chopped

Directions:

1. Put the watermelon slices in the plate in one layer. Then sprinkle them with blueberries, goat cheese, and fresh parsley.

Nutrition: Calories 69 Protein 4.4g Carbohydrates 1.4g Fat 5.1g

35. Sprouts Pizza

Preparation time: 15 minutes

Cooking time: 15 minutes

Servings: 6

Ingredients:

- 4 oz wheat flour, whole grain
- 2 tablespoons olive oil
- ¼ teaspoon baking powder
- 5 oz chicken fillet, boiled
- 2 oz Mozzarella cheese, shredded
- 1 tomato, chopped
- 2 oz bean sprouts

Directions:

1. Make the pizza crust: mix wheat flour, olive oil, baking powder, and knead the dough. Roll it up in the shape of pizza crust and transfer in the pizza mold.
2. Then sprinkle it with chopped tomato, shredded chicken, and Mozzarella. Bake the pizza at 365F for 15 minutes. Sprinkle the cooked pizza with bean sprouts and cut into servings.

Nutrition: Calories 184 Protein 11.9g Carbohydrates 15.6g Fat 8.2g

VEGETARIAN DISHES

36. Zucchini Garlic Fries

Preparation Time: 15 minutes

Cooking Time: 20 minutes

Servings: 6

Ingredients:

- ¼ tsp. garlic powder
- ½ cup almond flour
- 2 large egg whites, beaten
- 3 medium zucchinis, sliced into fry sticks
- Salt and pepper to taste

Directions:

1. Preheat oven to 400°F.
2. Mix all ingredients in a bowl until the zucchini fries are well coated.
3. Place fries on cookie sheet and spread evenly.
4. Put in oven and cook for 20 minutes.
5. Halfway through cooking time, stir fries.

Nutrition: Calories: 11; Carbs: 1.1g; Protein: 1.5g; Fat: 0.1g

37. Zucchini Pasta with Mango-Kiwi Sauce

Preparation Time: 5 minutes

Cooking Time: 20 minutes

Servings: 2

Ingredients:

- 1 tsp. dried herbs – optional
- ½ Cup Raw Kale leaves, shredded
- 2 small dried figs
- 3 medjool dates
- 4 medium kiwis
- 2 big mangos, seed discarded
- 2 cup zucchini, spiralized
- ¼ cup roasted cashew

Directions:

1. On a salad bowl, place kale then topped with zucchini noodles and sprinkle with dried herbs. Set aside.
2. In a food processor, grind to a powder the cashews. Add figs, dates, kiwis and mangoes then puree to a smooth consistency.
3. Pour over zucchini pasta, serve and enjoy.

Nutrition: Calories: 530; Carbs: 95.4g; Protein: 8.0g; Fat: 18.5g

FISH AND SEAFOOD

38. Baked Shrimp Mix

Preparation Time: 10 minutes

Cooking Time: 32 minutes

Servings: 4

Ingredients:

- 4 gold potatoes, peeled and sliced
- 2 fennel bulbs, trimmed and cut into wedges
- 2 shallots, chopped
- 2 garlic cloves, minced
- 3 tbsp. olive oil
- ½ cup kalamata olives, pitted and halved
- 2 lb. shrimp, peeled and deveined
- 1 tsp. lemon zest, grated
- 2 tsp. oregano, dried
- 4 oz. feta cheese, crumbled
- 2 tbsp. parsley, chopped

Directions:

1. In a roasting pan, combine the potatoes with 2 tbsp. oil, garlic and the rest of the ingredients except the shrimp, toss, introduce in the oven and bake at 450°F for 25 minutes.

2. Add the shrimp, toss, bake for 7 minutes more, divide between plates and serve.

Nutrition: Calories 341, Fat 19g, Fiber 9g, Carbs 34g, Protein 10g

39. Shrimp and Lemon Sauce

Preparation Time: 10 minutes

Cooking Time: 15 minutes

Servings: 4

Ingredients:

- 1 lb. shrimp, peeled and deveined
- 1/3 cup lemon juice
- 4 egg yolks
- 2 tbsp. olive oil
- 1 cup chicken stock
- Salt and black pepper to the taste
- 1 cup black olives, pitted and halved
- 1 tbsp. thyme, chopped

Directions:

1. In a bowl, mix the lemon juice with the egg yolks and whisk well.
2. Heat up a pan with the oil over medium heat, add the shrimp and cook for 2 minutes on each side and transfer to a plate.
3. Heat up a pan with the stock over medium heat, add some of this over the egg yolks and lemon juice mix and whisk well.
4. Add this over the rest of the stock, also add salt and pepper, whisk well and simmer for 2 minutes.

5. Add the shrimp and the rest of the ingredients, toss and serve right away.

Nutrition: Calories 237, Fat 15.3g, Fiber 4.6g, Carbs 15.4g, Protein 7.6g

40. Shrimp and Beans Salad

Preparation Time: 10 minutes

Cooking Time: 4 minutes

Servings: 4

Ingredients:

- 1 lb. shrimp, peeled and deveined
- 30 oz. canned cannellini beans, drained and rinsed
- 2 tbsp. olive oil
- 1 cup cherry tomatoes, halved
- 1 tsp. lemon zest, grated
- ½ cup red onion, chopped
- 4 handfuls baby arugula
- A pinch of salt and black pepper
- For the dressing:
- 3 tbsp. red wine vinegar
- 2 garlic cloves, minced
- ½ cup olive oil

Directions:

1. Heat up a pan with 2 tbsp. oil over medium-high heat, add the shrimp and cook for 2 minutes on each side.
2. In a salad bowl, combine the shrimp with the beans and the rest of the ingredients except the ones for the dressing and toss.
3. In a separate bowl, combine the vinegar with ½ cup oil and the garlic and whisk well.

4. Pour over the salad, toss and serve right away.

Nutrition: Calories 207, Fat 12.3g, Fiber 6.6g, Carbs 15.4g, Protein 8.7g

41. Pecan Salmon Fillets

Preparation Time: 10 minutes

Cooking Time: 15 minutes

Servings: 6

Ingredients:

- 3 tbsp. olive oil
- 3 tbsp. mustard
- 5 tsp. honey
- 1 cup pecans, chopped
- 6 salmon fillets, boneless
- 1 tbsp. lemon juice
- 3 tsp. parsley, chopped
- Salt and pepper to the taste

Directions:

1. In a bowl, mix the oil with the mustard and honey and whisk well.
2. Put the pecans and the parsley in another bowl.
3. Season the salmon fillets with salt and pepper, arrange them on a baking sheet lined with parchment paper, brush with the honey and mustard mix and top with the pecans mix.
4. Introduce in the oven at 400°F, bake for 15 minutes, divide between plates, drizzle the lemon juice on top and serve.

Nutrition: Calories 282, Fat 15.5g, Fiber 8.5g, Carbs 20.9g, Protein 16.8g

APPETIZER AND SNACK RECIPES

42. Smoky Loaded Eggplant Dip

Preparation time: 15 minutes

Cooking time: 20 minutes

Servings: 6

Ingredients:

- 1 large eggplant
- 1 ½ tablespoon Greek yoghurt
- 2 tablespoon tahini paste
- 1 garlic clove, chopped
- 1 tablespoon lemon juice
- 1 ½ teaspoon sumac
- ¾ teaspoon Aleppo pepper
- toasted pine nuts
- salt and pepper
- 1 tomato, diced
- ½ English cucumber, diced
- lemon juice
- parsley
- olive oil

Directions:

1. Add parsley, cucumber and tomato to a bowl. Season with ½ teaspoon sumac, salt and pepper. Add lemon juice and olive oil. Toss and set aside.
2. Turn a gas burner on high and turn eggplant on it every 5 minutes with a tong until charred and crispy, for 20 minutes. Remove from the heat and let cool.
3. Peel the skin off the eggplant and discard the stem. Transfer eggplant flesh to a colander and drain for 5 minutes.
4. Transfer flesh to a blender. Add yoghurt, tahini paste, garlic, lemon juice, salt, pepper, Aleppo pepper and sumac. Blend for 2 pulses to combine.
5. Transfer to a bowl. Cover and refrigerate for 30 minutes. Bring it to a room temperature and add olive oil on top. Add pine nuts. Add salad on top and serve.

Nutrition: Calories: 40 Carbs: 3g Fat: 4g Protein: 0g

43. Peanut Butter Banana Greek Yogurt Bowl

Preparation time: 15 minutes

Cooking time: 0 minutes

Servings: 4

Ingredients:

- 2 medium bananas, sliced
- 4 cups vanilla Greek yoghurt
- ¼ cup peanut butter
- 1 teaspoon nutmeg
- ¼ cup flax seed meal

Directions:

1. Divide the yoghurt equally among 4 bowls and add banana slices to it. Add peanut butter to a bowl and microwave for 40 seconds.
2. Add 1 tablespoon peanut butter over each bowl. Add nutmeg and flax seed meal to each bowl. Serve.

Nutrition: Calories: 110 Carbs: 13g Fat: 0g Protein: 15g

44. Roasted Chickpeas

Preparation time: 15 minutes

Cooking time: 30 minutes

Servings: 2

Ingredients:

- 2 tablespoons extra virgin olive oil
- 2 15 oz. cans chickpeas
- 2 teaspoon red wine vinegar
- 2 teaspoon lemon juice
- 1 teaspoon dried oregano
- ½ teaspoon garlic powder
- 1 teaspoon kosher salt
- ½ teaspoon black pepper, cracked

Directions:

1. Preheat the oven to 425F and line a baking sheet with parchment paper. Drain, rinse and dry chickpeas and put on a baking sheet.

2. Roast for 10 minutes, then remove from the oven. Turn chickpeas and roast for 10 minutes. Add the remaining ingredients to a bowl and mix well.

3. Add chickpeas to it and mix to coat well. Transfer coated chickpeas back to the oven and roast for 10 minutes. Cool completely. Serve.

Nutrition: Calories: 191 Carbs: 27g Fat: 1g Protein: 9g

45. Savory Feta Spinach and Sweet Red Pepper Muffins

Preparation time: 15 minutes

Cooking time: 25 minutes

Servings: 12

Ingredients:

- 2 eggs
- 2 ¾ cups all-purpose flour
- ¼ cup sugar
- 1 teaspoon paprika
- 2 teaspoons baking powder
- ¾ cup low-fat milk
- ½ cup extra virgin olive oil
- ¾ cup feta, crumbled
- 1/3 cup jarred florina peppers, drained and patted dry
- ¾ teaspoon salt
- 1 ¼ cup spinach, thinly sliced

Directions:

1. Preheat the oven to 375F. Mix sugar, flour, baking powder, paprika and salt in a bowl. Mix eggs, olive oil and milk in another bowl.
2. Add wet ingredients to dry and mix until blended. Add spinach, feta and peppers and mix well.
3. Line a muffin pan with liners and add the mixture to them equally. Bake for 25 minutes. Let cool for 10

minutes. Remove from the tray. Cool for 2 hours and serve.

Nutrition: Calories: 295 Carbs: 27g Fat: 18g Protein: 8g

DESSERT RECIPES

46. Lemon and Garlic Fettucine

Preparation Time: 5 Minutes

Cooking Time: 15 Minutes

Servings: 5

Ingredients:

- 8 ounces of whole wheat fettuccine
- 4 tablespoons of extra virgin olive oil
- 4 cloves of minced garlic
- 1 cup of fresh breadcrumbs
- ¼ cup of lemon juice
- 1 teaspoon of freshly ground pepper
- ½ teaspoon of salt
- 2 cans of 4 ounce boneless and skinless sardines (dipped in tomato sauce)
- ½ cup of chopped up fresh parsley
- ¼ cup of finely shredded Parmesan cheese

Directions:

1. Take a large-sized pot and bring water to a boil.
2. Cook pasta for 10 minutes until Al Dente.
3. Take a small-sized skillet and place it over medium heat.
4. Add 2 tablespoons of oil and allow it to heat up.

5. Add garlic and cook for 20 seconds.
6. Transfer the garlic to a medium-sized bowl
7. Add breadcrumbs to the hot skillet and cook for 5-6 minutes until golden
8. Whisk in lemon juice, pepper and salt into the garlic bowl
9. Add pasta to the bowl (with garlic) and sardines, parsley and Parmesan
10. Stir well and sprinkle bread crumbs
11. Enjoy!

Nutrition: Calories: 480 Fat: 21g Carbohydrates: 53g Protein: 23g

47. Roasted Broccoli with Parmesan

Preparation Time: 10 Minutes

Cooking Time: 10 Minutes

Servings: 4

Ingredients:

- 2 head broccolis, cut into florets
- 2 tablespoons extra-virgin olive oil
- 2 teaspoons garlic, minced
- Zest of 1 lemon
- Pinch of salt
- ½ cup Parmesan cheese, grated

Directions:

1. Pre-heat your oven to 400 degrees Fahrenheit.
2. Take a large bowl and add broccoli with 2 tablespoons olive oil, lemon zest, garlic, lemon juice and salt.
3. Spread mix on the baking sheet in single layer and sprinkle with Parmesan cheese.
4. Bake for 10 minutes until tender.
5. Transfer broccoli to serving the dish.
6. Serve and enjoy!

Nutrition: Calories: 154 Fat: 11g Carbohydrates: 10g Protein: 9g

48. Spinach and Feta Bread

Preparation Time: 10 Minutes

Cooking Time: 12 Minutes

Servings: 6

Ingredients:

- 6 ounces of sun-dried tomato pesto
- 6 pieces of 6-inch whole wheat pita bread
- 2 chopped up Roma plum tomatoes
- 1 bunch of rinsed and chopped spinach
- 4 sliced fresh mushrooms
- ½ cup of crumbled feta cheese
- 2 tablespoons of grated Parmesan cheese
- 3 tablespoons of olive oil
- Ground black pepper as needed

Directions:

1. Pre-heat your oven to 350 degrees Fahrenheit.
2. Spread your tomato pesto onto one side of your pita bread and place on your baking sheet (with the pesto side up).
3. Top up the pitas with spinach, tomatoes, feta cheese, mushrooms and Parmesan cheese.
4. Drizzle with some olive oil and season nicely with pepper.
5. Bake in your oven for around 12 minutes until the breads are crispy.

6. Cut up the pita into quarters and serve!

Nutrition: Calories: 350 Fat: 17g Carbohydrates: 41g Protein: 11g

49. Quick Zucchini Bowl

Preparation Time: 10 Minutes

Cooking Time: 10 Minutes

Servings: 4

Ingredients:

- ½ pound of pasta
- 2 tablespoons of olive oil
- 6 crushed garlic cloves
- 1 teaspoon of red chili
- 2 finely sliced spring onions
- 3 teaspoons of chopped rosemary
- 1 large zucchini cut up in half, lengthways and sliced
- 5 large portabella mushrooms
- 1 can of tomatoes
- 4 tablespoons of Parmesan cheese
- Fresh ground black pepper

Directions:

1. Cook the pasta.
2. Take a large-sized frying pan and place over medium heat.
3. Add oil and allow the oil to heat up.
4. Add garlic, onion and chili and sauté for a few minutes until golden.
5. Add zucchini, rosemary and mushroom and sauté for a few minutes.

6. Increase the heat to medium-high and add tinned tomatoes to the sauce until thick.
7. Drain your boiled pasta and transfer to a serving platter.
8. Pour the tomato mix on top and mix using tongs.
9. Garnish with Parmesan cheese and freshly ground black pepper.
10. Enjoy!

Nutrition: Calories: 361 Fat: 12g Carbohydrates: 47g Protein: 14g

50. Healthy Basil Platter

Preparation Time: 25 Minutes

Cooking Time: 15 Minutes

Servings: 4

Ingredients:

- 2 pieces of red pepper seeded and cut up into chunks
- 2 pieces of red onion cut up into wedges
- 2 mild red chilies, diced and seeded
- 3 coarsely chopped garlic cloves
- 1 teaspoon of golden caster sugar
- 2 tablespoons of olive oil (plus additional for serving)
- 2 pounds of small ripe tomatoes quartered up
- 12 ounces of dried pasta
- Just a handful of basil leaves
- 2 tablespoons of grated Parmesan

Directions:

1. Pre-heat the oven to 392 degrees Fahrenheit.
2. Take a large-sized roasting tin and scatter pepper, red onion, garlic and chilies.
3. Sprinkle sugar on top.
4. Drizzle olive oil then season with pepper and salt.
5. Roast the veggies in your oven for 15 minutes.
6. Take a large-sized pan and cook the pasta in boiling, salted water until Al Dente.
7. Drain them.

8. Remove the veggies from the oven and tip in the pasta into the veggies.

9. Toss well and tear basil leaves on top.

10. Sprinkle Parmesan and enjoy!

Nutrition: Calories: 452 Fat: 8g Carbohydrates: 88g Protein: 14g

51. Cucumber Sandwich Bites

Preparation Time: 5 minutes

Cooking Time: 0 minutes

Servings: 12

INGREDIENTS:

- 1 cucumber, sliced
- 8 slices whole wheat bread
- 2 tablespoons cream cheese, soft
- 1 tablespoon chives, chopped
- ¼ cup avocado, peeled, pitted and mashed
- 1 teaspoon mustard
- Salt and black pepper to the taste

DIRECTIONS:

1. Spread the mashed avocado on each bread slice, also spread the rest of the ingredients except the cucumber slices.
2. Divide the cucumber slices on the bread slices, cut each slice in thirds, arrange on a platter and serve as an appetizer.

NUTRITION: Calories 187 Fat 12.4g Carbohydrates 4.5g Protein 8.2g

52. Yogurt Dip

Preparation Time: 10 minutes

Cooking Time: 0 minutes

Servings: 6

INGREDIENTS:

- 2 cups Greek yogurt
- 2 tablespoons pistachios, toasted and chopped
- A pinch of salt and white pepper
- 2 tablespoons mint, chopped
- 1 tablespoon kalamata olives, pitted and chopped
- ¼ cup zaatar spice
- ¼ cup pomegranate seeds
- 1/3 cup olive oil

DIRECTIONS:

1. Mix the yogurt with the pistachios and the rest of the ingredients, whisk well, divide into small cups and serve with pita chips on the side.

NUTRITION: Calories 294 Fat 18g Carbohydrates 2g Protein 10g

53. Tomato Bruschetta

Preparation Time: 10 minutes

Cooking Time: 10 minutes

Servings: 6

INGREDIENTS:

- 1 baguette, sliced
- 1/3 cup basil, chopped
- 6 tomatoes, cubed
- 2 garlic cloves, minced
- A pinch of salt and black pepper
- 1 teaspoon olive oil
- 1 tablespoon balsamic vinegar
- ½ teaspoon garlic powder
- Cooking spray

DIRECTIONS:

1. Situate the baguette slices on a baking sheet lined with parchment paper, grease with cooking spray. Bake for 10 minutes at 400 degrees.

2. Combine the tomatoes with the basil and the remaining ingredients, toss well and leave aside for 10 minutes. Divide the tomato mix on each baguette slice, arrange them all on a platter and serve.

NUTRITION: Calories 162 Fat 4g Carbohydrates 29g Protein 4g

54. Olives and Cheese Stuffed Tomatoes

Preparation Time: 10 minutes

Cooking Time: 0 minutes

Servings: 24

INGREDIENTS:

- 24 cherry tomatoes, top cut off and insides scooped out
- 2 tablespoons olive oil
- ¼ teaspoon red pepper flakes
- ½ cup feta cheese, crumbled
- 2 tablespoons black olive paste
- ¼ cup mint, torn

DIRECTIONS:

1. In a bowl, mix the olives paste with the rest of the ingredients except the cherry tomatoes and whisk well. Stuff the cherry tomatoes with this mix, arrange them all on a platter and serve as an appetizer.

NUTRITION: Calories 136 Fat 8.6g Carbohydrates 5.6g Protein 5.1g

55. Pepper Tapenade

Preparation Time: 10 minutes

Cooking Time: 0 minutes

Servings: 4

INGREDIENTS:

- 7 ounces roasted red peppers, chopped
- ½ cup parmesan, grated
- 1/3 cup parsley, chopped
- 14 ounces canned artichokes, drained and chopped
- 3 tablespoons olive oil
- ¼ cup capers, drained
- 1 and ½ tablespoons lemon juice
- 2 garlic cloves, minced

DIRECTIONS:

1. In your blender, combine the red peppers with the parmesan and the rest of the ingredients and pulse well. Divide into cups and serve as a snack.

NUTRITION: Calories 200 Fat 5.6g Carbohydrates 12.4g Protein 4.6g

56. Coriander Falafel

Preparation Time: 10 minutes

Cooking Time: 10 minutes

Servings: 8

INGREDIENTS:

- 1 cup canned garbanzo beans
- 1 bunch parsley leaves
- 1 yellow onion, chopped
- 5 garlic cloves, minced
- 1 teaspoon coriander, ground
- A pinch of salt and black pepper
- ¼ teaspoon cayenne pepper
- ¼ teaspoon baking soda
- ¼ teaspoon cumin powder
- 1 teaspoon lemon juice
- 3 tablespoons tapioca flour
- Olive oil for frying

DIRECTIONS:

1. In your food processor, combine the beans with the parsley, onion and the rest the ingredients except the oil and the flour and pulse well.
2. Transfer the mix to a bowl, add the flour, stir well, shape 16 balls out of this mix and flatten them a bit.
3. Preheat pan over medium-high heat, add the falafels, cook them for 5 minutes on both sides, put in paper

towels, drain excess grease, arrange them on a platter and serve as an appetizer.

NUTRITION: Calories 122 Fat 6.2g Carbohydrates 12.3g Protein 3.1g

57. Red Pepper Hummus

Preparation Time: 10 minutes

Cooking Time: 0 minutes

Servings: 6

INGREDIENTS:

- 6 ounces roasted red peppers, peeled and chopped
- 16 ounces canned chickpeas, drained and rinsed
- ¼ cup Greek yogurt
- 3 tablespoons tahini paste
- Juice of 1 lemon
- 3 garlic cloves, minced
- 1 tablespoon olive oil
- A pinch of salt and black pepper
- 1 tablespoon parsley, chopped

DIRECTIONS:

1. In your food processor, combine the red peppers with the rest of the ingredients except the oil and the parsley and pulse well. Add the oil, pulse again, divide into cups, sprinkle the parsley on top and serve as a party spread.

NUTRITION: Calories 255 Fat 11.4g Carbohydrates 17.4g Protein 6.5g

58. White Bean Dip

Preparation Time: 10 minutes

Cooking Time: 0 minutes

Servings: 4

INGREDIENTS:

- 15 ounces canned white beans, drained and rinsed
- 6 ounces canned artichoke hearts, drained and quartered
- 4 garlic cloves, minced
- 1 tablespoon basil, chopped
- 2 tablespoons olive oil
- Juice of ½ lemon
- Zest of ½ lemon, grated
- Salt and black pepper to the taste

DIRECTIONS:

1. In your food processor, combine the beans with the artichokes and the rest of the ingredients except the oil and pulse well. Add the oil gradually, pulse the mix again, divide into cups and serve as a party dip.

NUTRITION: Calories 27 Fat 11.7g Carbohydrates 18.5g Protein 16.5g

59. Hummus with Ground Lamb

Preparation Time: 10 minutes

Cooking Time: 15 minutes

Servings: 8

INGREDIENTS:

- 10 ounces hummus
- 12 ounces lamb meat, ground
- ½ cup pomegranate seeds
- ¼ cup parsley, chopped
- 1 tablespoon olive oil
- Pita chips for serving

DIRECTIONS:

1. Preheat pan over medium-high heat, cook the meat, and brown for 15 minutes stirring often. Spread the hummus on a platter, spread the ground lamb all over, also spread the pomegranate seeds and the parsley and serve with pita chips as a snack.

NUTRITION: Calories 133 Fat 9.7g Carbohydrates 6.4g Protein 5.4g

60. Eggplant Dip

Preparation Time: 10 minutes

Cooking Time: 40 minutes

Servings: 4

INGREDIENTS:

- 1 eggplant, poked with a fork
- 2 tablespoons tahini paste
- 2 tablespoons lemon juice
- 2 garlic cloves, minced
- 1 tablespoon olive oil
- Salt and black pepper to the taste
- 1 tablespoon parsley, chopped

DIRECTIONS:

1. Put the eggplant in a roasting pan, bake at 400 degrees F for 40 minutes, cool down, peel and transfer to your food processor.
2. Blend the rest of the ingredients except the parsley, pulse well, divide into small bowls and serve as an appetizer with the parsley sprinkled on top.

NUTRITION: Calories 121 Fat 4.3g Carbohydrates 1.4g Protein 4.3g

9 781802 155